WHAT'S WRONG WITH MY
STOMACH?

*Understanding Digestive System Disorders and What You Can Do
To Repair Your System Naturally*

**BY INVESTIGATIVE REPORTER
GREGORY CIOLA**

This page is left intentionally blank

Table of Contents

Disclaimer

This book is not intended to provide medical advice or take the place of medical advice and treatment recommended by your physician or health care provider. This book is published for the express purpose of sharing educational information, scientific and medical research, nutritional knowledge, and opinions gathered from the author's own investigations. Readers are advised to consult their medical doctor or qualified health care professional regarding the treatment options for their diagnosed condition. If you have a medical related condition or are taking prescription medications, you should consult with your physician before taking any alternative approaches.

We do not advise anyone to discontinue medical treatment or to begin a supplementation program without the proper supervision of a health care professional. Should you choose to make use of the information contained herein without first consulting a health care professional, you are prescribing for yourself, which is your Constitutional and Divine right. However, neither the author, nor the publisher assumes any responsibility for the decisions you make based upon reading this book.

Copyright © 2018 Investigator's Report

Address all correspondence to:

Investigator's Report

13506 Summerport Village Pkwy #314

Windermere, FL 34786

Toll Free: 800.593.6273

Local: 828.357.5155

Fax: 407.798.7731

Website: www.investigatorsreport.com

Email: editor@investigatorsreport.com

"A good eater must be a good man; for a good eater must have a good digestion, and a good digestion depends upon a good conscience."
– **Benjamin Disraeli, 'The Young Duke' (1831)**

"If people let the government decide what foods they eat and what medicines they take, their bodies will soon be in as sorry a state as are the souls of those who live under tyranny." — **Thomas Jefferson**

"The doctor of the future will give little medicine but will interest his patients in the care of the human frame, diet, and in the cause and prevention of disease." — **Thomas A. Edison**

Chapter 1

GI DISORDERS HAVE BECOME THE MOST COMMON HEALTH PROBLEMS AFFLICITNG AMERICANS ACCORDING TO GOVERNMENT STATISTICS

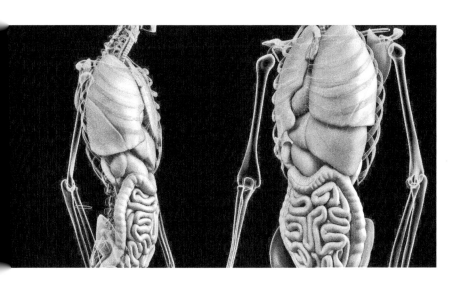

A Fox News survey published in 2013 reported that 74% of the respondents are living with GI discomfort.

"Over half of them never discussed it with their doctor," said Dr. Rashini Raj, a gastroenterologist at NYU Langone Medical Center in New York City, on behalf of AbbVie Pharmaceuticals, who commissioned the survey. "And that's probably the most alarming part for me, because as you know, sometimes this can be a sign of a more serious underlying condition: celiac disease, Crohn's disease, EPI or exocrine pancreatic insufficiency -- so these are symptoms you shouldn't ignore, and, unfortunately, a lot of people don't feel comfortable talking about them." [i]

That last sentence says a mouthful. People don't feel comfortable talking about them. It's embarrassing. As a result, they live in distress and suffer through their troubles while remaining silent. That likely means that the real statistics are much higher.

What is happening?

How is it that so many people are suddenly dealing with digestive conditions?

Our society used to think this only happened to older adults when their health started failing later in life. That's not the case anymore. One of the most significant segments of the population dealing with digestive issues is children. Gluten sensitivity, IBS, constipation, and allergies to dairy, nuts, and fish have become epidemic in children.

Without proper digestion, you are a candidate for many serious diseases. A good analogy would be to compare digestion to a warning light on your car's dashboard. The light on your panel comes on blinking, "service engine." You know that you must take the car to a dealer or repair shop immediately. Left unchecked, it could be a sign of something much more severe, and there's a good chance your car will stop running if you ignore the warning.

Consider any digestive related condition a warning light. "Service body." If you fail to heed the warning, your body can fail. Sadly, out of either fear or lack of understanding, a significant percentage of the population does nothing.

I was somewhat shocked when I learned that intestinal disorders had become the number one complaint to doctors and the leading cause of hospitalizations. That's why I have written this book. People are hungry for answers, and they need to understand that they are not alone.

Most people would probably think that cancer, diabetes, or cardiovascular issues would top the list of doctor visits. When I talk about digestion, I realize that this is a vast subject. It can include constipation, IBS, Crohn's disease, ulcerative colitis, inflammatory bowel, leaky gut, diverticulitis, GERD, infections, hemorrhoids, bloating, gas, bad breath, mucus build-up, stomach pains, digestive complications, flora degradation, weakened immunity, and many other related conditions. Some gastrointestinal diseases are acute, lasting only a short time, while others are chronic, or long-lasting.

This book is not intended to be a dissertation on every single digestive condition afflicting humanity. I hope to give you a general overview of gastrointestinal diseases and what is causing them, and then leave you with some simple solutions that can help you fix your problems and get your health back. I will dial in a little bit more on some of the more common digestive conditions in the next chapter.

If chronic constipation is your problem, it can lead to the slow accumulation of toxins and fecal debris in the digestive system that can fester and stew into a more serious problem if left untreated. This waste can become a food source for microbial scavengers such as parasites. Digestive toxins can bombard the body with free radicals and interfere with cellular integrity. A backed up digestive system will also hinder nutrients from making their way into the bloodstream causing deficiencies. It is impossible to overcome the escalating prevalence of disease or restore ailing health without focusing on maintaining a smooth-running digestive system.

Filling up on processed and packaged foods, fried foods and a lot of meat every day year after year takes a toll on the body. Despite the apparent move towards better health in America, the fact is very few are doing what it takes to avoid the health-destroying landmines. The grocery stores shelves are jam-packed with junk food that will turn the average person's intestinal system into the plaster of Paris. The fast-food restaurant business is booming for two simple reasons – it's cheap, and it's convenient. Most of what gets passed off as healthy on packaging and labels is a total scam.

To top it off, just about everyone is ingesting residues of Roundup (glyphosate) and GMOs which have been proven to disrupt digestive health. Add on the hundreds of chemicals you're probably consuming in municipal water and bottled drinks, and it's no wonder why these problems have become so prevalent.

This dangerous yet common lifestyle can lead to a bloated stomach, weight gain, stomach pain, living on antacids, and suffering from severe constipation. In most instances, it's a toxic, congested, malfunctioning digestive system that leads to the other filtration organs becoming weakened and overburdened.

If you look at the anatomy of the digestive system pictured above, it's apparent that it's all connected like a well-weaved spider web. Medical science treats the human body as though it consists of a bunch of separate car parts and when something goes wrong you visit a specialist for that organ or system instead of a doctor that understands the complete picture.

When the colon is compacted and filled with toxins, constipation will lead to putrefactive protein, unhealthy fats, and fermented carbohydrates. This leads to the manufacturing of cancer-causing agents like isopropyl alcohol, hydroxyl free radicals, purines, ammonia, parasites, and germs, which will leak into the bloodstream and trigger a chain reaction of cell damage.

An impaired intestinal system can cause a person to have a stagnant, dirty, low oxygenated environment that is a breeding ground for bacteria, viruses, parasites, tapeworms, fungus, and eventually cancer. The human body can only withstand so much before there are consequences.

Chapter 2

A CLOSER LOOK AT SOME OF THE MORE COMMON DIGESTIVE DISORDERS

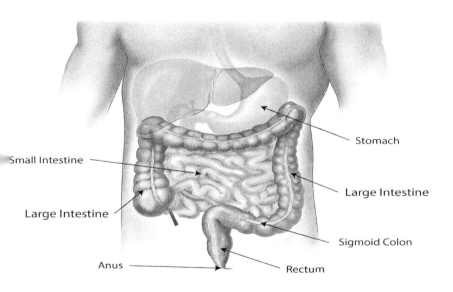

M any disorders affect the colon's ability to work properly. Some of the more common ones include:

- Polyps - extra tissue growing in the colon that can be come cancerous
- Ulcerative Colitis - ulcers of the colon and rectum
- Diverticulitis - inflammation or infection of pouches in the colon
- Irritable Bowel Syndrome (IBS) - an uncomfortable condition causing abdominal cramping and other symptoms
- Chronic Constipation
- Leaky Gut
- Acid Reflux (GERD)
- Acid Indigestion
- Stomach Pain
- Colorectal Cancer

Here are some alarming statistics provided by the US Department of Health and Human Services National Institute of Diabetes and Digestive and Kidney Diseases.

All Digestive Diseases

Prevalence: 60 to 70 million people affected by all digestive diseases

Ambulatory care visits: 48.3 million (2010)

Primary diagnosis at office visits: 36.6 million (2010)

Primary diagnosis at emergency department visits: 7.9 million (2010)

Primary diagnosis at outpatient department visits: 3.8 million (2010)

Hospitalizations: 21.7 million (2010)

Mortality: 245,921 deaths (2009)

Diagnostic and therapeutic inpatient procedures: 5.4 million—12 percent of all inpatient procedures (2007)

Ambulatory surgical procedures: 20.4 million—20 percent of all "write-in" surgical procedures (2010) [ii]

CONSTIPATION

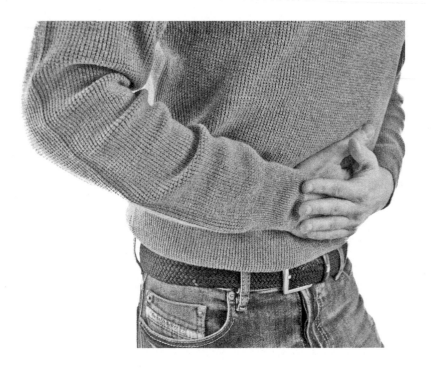

The US NIH considers constipation to be a condition in which you typically have:

- fewer than three bowel movements a week and
- bowel movements with stools that are hard, dry, and small, making them painful or difficult to pass

Constipation is one of the most common gastrointestinal (GI) problems, affecting about 42 million people in the United States.[iii] Treatments for constipation include making changes in your eating, diet, and nutrition; exercise and lifestyle changes; medicines and supplements; biofeedback; and surgery.

What causes constipation?

Constipation can happen for many reasons, and constipation may have more than one cause at a time. Among the most common causes of constipation are:

- slow movement of stool through the colon
- delayed emptying of the colon from pelvic disorders, especially in women
- a form of irritable bowel syndrome (IBS) that has symptoms of both IBS and constipation, also called IBS with constipation, or IBS-C.[iv]

Other things that can cause constipation include diets low in fiber, lack of physical activity, sitting all day without exercise, and insufficient water intake. Medications such as antacids, anticholinergics, anticonvulsants, antispasmodics, calcium channel blockers, diuretics, iron supplements, narcotics, tumors, inflammation, traveling, pregnancy, and ignoring the urge to have a bowel movement are other contributors.

The Importance of Fiber for Constipation

Despite the advantages, Americans do not consume the maximum amount fiber as they should. There are two forms of fiber, soluble and insoluble, which can be used to treat and stop constipation. Both types of fiber are essential for keeping the intestinal system running smoothly.

Soluble fiber permits additional water to stay in your stool, making waste softer, more substantial, and thus easier to pass through the intestines. Insoluble fiber adds bulk to your fecal material that hastens its passage through your gut and prevents that constipated feeling. Those who eat a diet high in fiber are less likely to become constipated.

The simplest way to get additional fiber in your diet is through food. Feeding on foods rich in fiber can maximize your intake of many different nutrients. When adding fiber to your diet, it's important to start slowly, so you don't experience gas pains. Increasing fiber over time can offer your body time to regulate. Getting enough fiber can help you have healthy bowel movements and forestall constipation.

Beta Glucan and Digestive Health

A unique form of fiber that is often overlooked is beta glucan. Beta-glucan is proven to be naturally useful in helping to manage weight, blood sugar and cholesterol - all factors associated with diabetes, heart disease, obesity and immune system related issues.

"Beta-glucan (β-glucan) is a soluble fiber readily available from oat and barley grains that has been gaining interest due to its multiple functional and bioactive properties. Its beneficial role in insulin resistance, dyslipidemia, hypertension, and obesity is being continuously documented. The fermentability of β-glucans and their ability to form highly viscous solutions in the human gut may constitute the basis of their health benefits. Consequently, the applicability of β-glucan as a food ingredient is being widely considered with the dual purposes of increasing the fiber content of food products and enhancing their health properties." [v]

Unlike starch and sugar, intestinal enzymes do not digest beta-glucan. Instead, beta-glucan transforms into a water-soluble, non-digestible gel. This gel:

- Coats the intestines

- Traps carbohydrates and dietary fat

- Slows the rate of digestion

- Assists the body with nutrient absorption

- Helps eliminate fats and cholesterol

ACID INDIGESTION, ACID REFLUX AND GERD

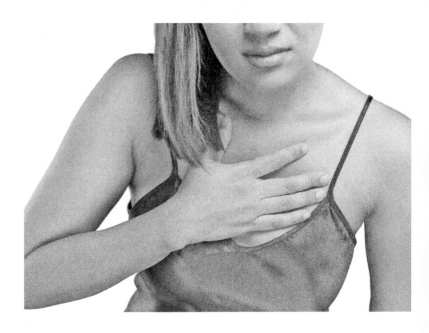

Gastroesophageal reflux (GER) happens when your stomach contents come back up into your esophagus causing heartburn (also called acid reflux). Gastroesophageal reflux disease (GERD) is a long-lasting and more serious form of GER.

Symptoms & Causes

The most common symptom of gastroesophageal reflux disease (GERD) is persistent heartburn, also called acid reflux. GERD happens when your lower esophageal sphincter becomes weak or relaxes when it shouldn't.

Diagnosis

Your doctor diagnoses gastroesophageal reflux (GER) and gastroesophageal reflux disease (GERD) by reviewing your symptoms and medical history. If your heartburn or other symptoms don't improve with lifestyle changes and medication, you may need testing.

You can reduce your gastroesophageal reflux disease (GERD) symptoms by changing your diet and avoiding foods and drinks that make your symptoms worse.[vi]

Food and dietary habits that are linked to acid reflux include:

- Consuming chocolate, carbonated drinks, and acidic juices
- Eating larger meals
- A high intake of table salt
- A diet low in dietary fiber
- Alcohol

- Lying down within 2 to 3 hours of eating a meal
- Caffeine

Other factors that may trigger acid reflux include being overweight, taking certain medications, smoking, pregnancy, hiatal hernia, previous surgery and preexisting health conditions. Important lifestyle tips that may help prevent acid reflux include:

- Getting plenty of exercise
- Maintaining a healthy weight
- Quitting smoking
- Drinking plenty of water
- Natural remedies: diet and nutrition

LEAKY GUT

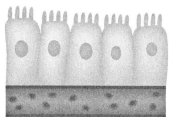
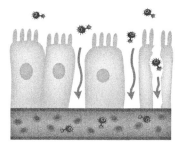

Normal Tight Junction   Leaky and Inflamed

A common disorder that develops when lesions form in the intestinal lining. These lesions have abnormally large spaces between the cell walls, allowing toxic material to seep into the bloodstream. Autism, rheumatoid arthritis, periodontal disease, chronic fatigue syndrome, Crohn's disease, and colitis all stem from the inflammation triggered by a leaky gut. Conditions such as small intestinal bacterial overgrowth (SIBO) and Irritable Bowel Syndrome (IBS) are a few examples of conditions that may cause leaky gut. Malabsorption of nutrients, candida and parasitic infections along with food sensitivities and allergies are conditions associated with a leaky gut. Inflammatory skin conditions like eczema, psoriasis and acne indicate a leaky gut too. The US NIH reports the following about leaky gut.

"The intestinal epithelial lining, together with factors secreted from it, forms a barrier that separates the host from the environment. In pathologic conditions, the permeability of the epithelial lining may be compromised allowing the passage of toxins, antigens, and bacteria in the lumen to enter the blood stream creating a 'leaky gut.' In individuals with a genetic predisposition, a leaky gut may allow environmental factors to enter the body and trigger the initiation and development of autoimmune disease. Growing evidence shows that the gut microbiota is important in supporting the epithelial barrier and therefore plays a key role in the regulation of environmental factors that enter the body. Several recent reports have shown that probiotics can reverse the leaky gut by enhancing the production of tight junction proteins;

however, additional and longer-term studies are still required. Conversely, pathogenic bacteria that can facilitate a leaky gut and induce autoimmune symptoms can be ameliorated with the use of antibiotic treatment. Therefore, it is hypothesized that modulating the gut microbiota can serve as a potential method for regulating intestinal permeability and may help to alter the course of autoimmune diseases in susceptible individuals." [vii]

Chapter 3

INTESTINAL LANDMINE #1:

OVERUSE OF ANTIBIOTICS

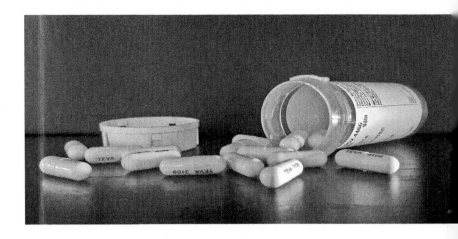

O veruse of antibiotics is a primary source of gastrointestinal problems. Antibiotics are not selective; they target and kill both good and bad bacteria in the digestive system. Antibiotics damage your body's microflora and intestinal ecology. If you have ever used antibiotics it is essential to take steps to rebuild healthy gut flora through a proper diet and supplementation with probiotics. If you have never done this after a round of antibiotics, or if you have been on long-term use of antibiotics, you are more than likely suffering from digestive distress syndrome.

You may be that unique person who hasn't taken antibiotics, or you followed through with probiotic supplementation after taking them. However, very few consider that our food supply is a significant source of antibiotic exposure. Let's face it; we are barraged with antibiotics. The most substantial purchasers of antibiotics are farmers. They treat most of the conventional farm animals raised for food with them. Then we have all the antibacterial soaps with triclosan to contend with as well.

"It is ironic that this humbled fungus, hailed as a benefactor of mankind, may by its very success prove to be a deciding factor in the decline of the present civilization." - Dr. John I. Pitt, The Genus

Penicillium, Academic Press, 1979

Our society has become conditioned to think that at the first sign of a sniffle, sore throat or a cough that you must run to the doctor as though they are the high priests of medicine with all the answers. The routine is SOP (standard operating procedure). You walk in, tell them your symptoms, they run a few quick tests, look in your ears and down your throat and send you on your way with a prescription.

How many patients question how this will affect their digestive system?

Are there long-term consequences?

The US NIH states the following in one report posted on their website:

"In addition to the development of resistance, the use of antibiotics heavily disrupts the ecology of the human microbiome (i.e., the collection of cells, genes, and metabolites from the bacteria, eukaryotes, and viruses that inhabit the human body). A dysbiotic microbiome may

INVESTIGATOR'S REPORT

not perform vital functions such as nutrient supply, vitamin produc-
tion, and protection from pathogens. Dysbiosis of the microbiome has
been associated with a large number of health problems and causally
implicated in metabolic, immunological, and developmental disorders,
as well as susceptibility to development of infectious diseases. The
wide variety of systems involved in these diseases provides ample cause
for concern over the unintentional consequences of antibiotic use."[viii]

FLORA'S #1 ENEMY - ANTIBIOTICS!

Intestinal flora (probiotics) are colonies of life generating microscopic bacteria found in both the small and large intestine. Flora serves as the intestinal system's clean-up crew and is also responsible for synthesizing a wide variety of nutrients in a manner that is similar to how microbes in the soil function with plants. The definition of "aerobic" is anything that pertains to or is caused by the presence of oxygen. Anything anaerobic either lacks oxygen or destroys oxygen. With probiotics, I am referring to life-giving oxygen-producing bacteria.

While probiotic means to be in favor of life, antibiotic has the exact opposite meaning. "Anti" means to be against something. In other words, antibiotics by their very name and nature are counterproductive to life. Most antibiotics cannot distinguish between good and bad germs. Antibiotics can kill everything. Excessive use of antibiotics will cause havoc on your digestive system, which then has a cascading domino effect on your entire health. Doctors have overprescribed antibiotics for decades, and very few people who use them even understand the importance of rebuilding healthy intestinal flora after taking them.

Many common health problems are directly attributed to the overuse of antibiotics. Sadly, in their lack of understanding on how the human body functions, doctors are prescribing antibiotics like they're handing out candy. We need to question medical intervention a little further before putting things into our body that can potentially harm it. There are plenty of safe, natural alternatives such as colloidal silver, herbs, minerals and essential oils that can do amazing things for fighting infections without harming your body's delicate flora balance.

The US NIH reports the following on the connection between healthy flora and digestive function.

"Gut bacteria are an important component of the microbiota ecosystem in the human gut, which is colonized by 1014 microbes,

ten times more than the human cells. Gut bacteria play an important role in human health, such as supplying essential nutrients, synthesizing vitamin K, aiding in the digestion of cellulose, and promoting angiogenesis and enteric nerve function. However, they can also be potentially harmful due to the change of their composition when the gut ecosystem undergoes abnormal changes in the light of the use of antibiotics, illness, stress, aging, bad dietary habits, and lifestyle. Dysbiosis of the gut bacteria communities can cause many chronic diseases, such as inflammatory bowel disease, obesity, cancer, and autism." [ix]

Chapter 4

INTESTINAL LANDMINE #2:

ROUNDUP (GLYPHOSATE)

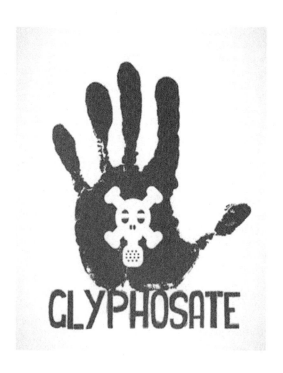

INVESTIGATOR'S REPORT

G lyphosate, the active chemical in Roundup that is sprayed on a huge percentage of our crops and consumed as a by-product of modern farming by millions of Americans every day, has been proven to cause all sorts of gastrointestinal disorders that are linked to our current disease epidemic. Our own US National Institutes of Health (US NIH) has an incredible report posted on their website that outlines the areas in the body that glyphosate is known to cause problems. Ironically, most of them deal with the intestinal system. There are also significant associations with glyphosate causing mineral depletion and imbalances. Glyphosate is linked to gluten intolerance, celiac disease, inflammatory bowel disease, disruption of enzymes, interference of gut bacteria, diarrhea, skin rashes, among many other things. This study is the smoking gun that should put Monsanto on the hot seat.

Here is a highlight of the study, however, you should go online and read the entire report which nails Roundup as being one of the main contributors to an intestinal apocalypse.

Glyphosate is the active ingredient in the herbicide Roundup. It is a broad-spectrum herbicide, considered to be nearly nontoxic to humans (Williams et al., 2000). However, a recent paper (Samsel & Seneff, 2013), argued that glyphosate may be a key contributor to the obesity epidemic and the autism epidemic in the United States, as well as to several other diseases and conditions, such as Alzheimer's disease, Parkinson's disease, infertility, depression, and cancer. Glyphosate suppresses 5-enolpyruvylshikimic acid-3-phosphate synthase (EPSP synthase), the rate-limiting step in the synthesis of the aromatic amino acids, tryptophan, tyrosine, and phenylalanine, in the shikimate pathway of bacteria, archaea and plants (de María et al., 1996). In plants, aromatic amino acids collectively represent up to 35% of the plant dry mass (Franz, 1997). This mode of action is unique to glyphosate among all emergent herbicides. *Humans do not possess this pathway, and therefore we depend upon our ingested food and our gut microbes to provide these essential nutrients. Glyphosate, patented as an antimicrobial (Monsanto Technology LLC, 2010), has been shown to disrupt gut bacteria in animals, preferentially killing beneficial forms and causing an overgrowth of pathogens*. Two other properties of glyphosate also negatively impact human health – chelation of minerals such as iron and cobalt, and interference with cytochrome P450 (CYP) enzymes, which play many important roles in the body. We will have much more to say about these aspects in later sections of this paper.

A recent study on glyphosate exposure in carnivorous fish

revealed *remarkable adverse effects throughout the digestive system* (Senapati et al., 2009). The activity of protease, lipase, and amylase were all decreased in the esophagus, stomach, and intestine of these fish following exposure to glyphosate. The authors also observed "disruption of mucosal folds and disarray of microvilli structure" in the intestinal wall, along with an exaggerated secretion of mucin throughout the alimentary tract. These features are highly reminiscent of celiac disease. Gluten peptides in wheat are hydrophobic and, therefore, resistant to degradation by gastric, pancreatic and intestinal proteases (Hershko & Patz, 2008). *Thus, the evidence from this effect on fish suggests that glyphosate may interfere with the breakdown of complex proteins in the human stomach, leaving larger fragments of wheat in the human gut that will then trigger an autoimmune response, leading to the defects in the lining of the small intestine that are characteristic of these fish exposed to glyphosate and of celiac patients.* As illustrated in Figure 1, the usage of glyphosate on wheat in the U.S. has risen sharply in the last decade, in step with the sharp rise in the incidence of Celiac disease. We explain the reasons for increased application of glyphosate to wheat in Section 13.[x]

Unless your diet consists entirely of 100% certified organic foods, there is no possible way you can, or are avoiding exposure to glyphosate. There are Very few farmers left that aren't using Roundup unless they are raising crops 100% organically. The simple fact is almost every single person in North America is ingesting glyphosate residues from their foods on a regular basis. It's no co-incidence that intestinal disorders are the number one complaint to doctors and the most prominent reason people are seeking out medical attention. Digestive related medical conditions are an epidemic, and it is a guaranteed recipe for some type of disease in your body if not corrected.

NaturalNews.com published an article in January 2018 that refers to a recent study conducted on glyphosate that supports it causing digestive problems.

"The latest study was carried out by a team led by Professor Gilles-Eric Seralini of the University of Caen. The study looked at fecal samples taken from rats and assessed their gut microbiomes. They found that female rats experienced significant changes in the presence of Roundup regardless of the dose to which they were exposed. It also damages the microbial activity of soil.

The researchers suggest that glyphosate use could be behind the recent spike in gut disease noted in industrialized nations that genetic reasons alone have failed to explain.

Of course, Roundup is not 100 percent glyphosate, so experts believe it could be worthwhile to repeat the study using a bigger group of animals to compare the effects of exposure to glyphosate alone as well as Roundup. It's possible that other ingredients in Roundup like adjuvants could be making this effect even more pronounced.

In fact, in regulatory evaluations of pesticides, it is only glyphosate in its isolated form that is tested for long-term safety, which means that calculations of safe levels are inherently inaccurate.

Professor Seralini said: 'The acceptable levels of glyphosate residues in food and drinks should be divided immediately by a factor of at least 1,000 because of these hidden poisons.'" [xi]

CELIAC DISEASE LINKED TO GLYPHOSATE

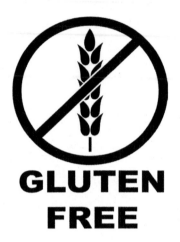

GLUTEN
FREE

The following information comes from the US NIH and is a blistering indictment by our own government of glyphosate and its link to Celiac disease.

"Celiac disease, and, more generally, gluten intolerance, is a growing problem worldwide, but especially in North America and Europe, where an estimated 5% of the population now suffers from it. Symptoms include nausea, diarrhea, skin rashes, macrocytic anemia and depression. It is a multifactorial disease associated with numerous nutritional deficiencies as well as reproductive issues and increased risk to thyroid disease, kidney failure and cancer. Here, we propose that glyphosate, the active ingredient in the herbicide, Roundup®, is the most important causal factor in this epidemic. Fish exposed to glyphosate develop digestive

problems that are reminiscent of celiac disease. Celiac disease is associ-ated with imbalances in gut bacteria that can be fully explained by the known effects of glyphosate on gut bacteria. Characteristics of celiac disease point to impairment in many cytochrome P450 enzymes, which are involved with detoxifying environmental toxins, activating vitamin D3, catabolizing vitamin A, and maintaining bile acid production and sulfate supplies to the gut. Glyphosate is known to inhibit cytochrome P450 enzymes. Deficiencies in iron, cobalt, molybdenum, copper and other rare metals associated with celiac disease can be attributed to glyphosate's strong ability to chelate these elements. Deficiencies in tryp-tophan, tyrosine, methionine and selenomethionine associated with celiac disease match glyphosate's known depletion of these amino acids. Celiac disease patients have an increased risk to non-Hodgkin's lymphoma, which has also been implicated in glyphosate exposure. Reproductive issues associated with celiac disease, such as infertility, miscarriages, and birth defects, can also be explained by glyphosate. Glyphosate residues in wheat and other crops are likely increasing recently due to the growing practice of crop desiccation just prior to the harvest. We argue that the practice of "ripening" sugar cane with glyphosate may explain the recent surge in kidney failure among agricultural workers in Central America. We conclude with a plea to governments to reconsider policies regarding the safety of glyphosate residues in foods." [xii]

INVESTIGATOR'S REPORT

Chapter 5

INTESTINAL LANDMINE #3:

GENETICALLY MODIFIED FOODS (GMOs)

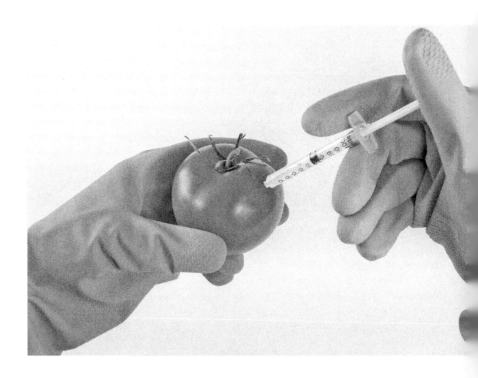

INVESTIGATOR'S REPORT

G enetically modified foods make up approximately 70-80% of all of the canned and packaged foods sold in the supermarket. Here's a good rule of thumb. Any food label that lists soy, cotton, canola, corn, beets, zucchini, yellow squash, or Hawaiian papaya that isn't organic or bears a seal from the Certified Non-GMO Project has likely been genetically engineered. While glyphosate is a pesticide sprayed on millions of acres of farmlands throughout America, including both conventionally grown and genetically engineered, biotechnology made the situation even worse. By altering the DNA of modern food crops and introducing a gene trait right into the plant itself, it has turned them into pesticide breeding factories. Glyphosate is terrible enough, but we also have to contend with GMO corn and cotton that has been altered with a bacterium called Bt (Bacillus thuringiensis). Monsanto got this product approved by claiming none of the bacteria would make its way past the human digestive system or cause digestive problems. Sadly, this turned out to be another big fat Monsanto lie just like many other claims they've made.

In a story by The Institute For Responsible Technology, they reported the following:

"Doctors at Sherbrooke University Hospital in Quebec found the corn's Bt-toxin in the blood of pregnant women and their babies, as well as in non-pregnant women. (Specifically, the toxin was identified in 93% of 30 pregnant women, 80% of umbilical blood in their babies, and 67% of 39 non-pregnant women.) The study has been accepted for publication in the peer reviewed journal Reproductive Toxicology….

There's already plenty of evidence that the Bt-toxin produced in GM corn and cotton plants is toxic to humans and mammals and triggers immune system responses. The fact that it flows through our blood supply, and that t passes through the placenta into fetuses, may help explain the rise in many disorders in the US since Bt crop varieties were first introduced in 1996…

Bt-toxin breaks open the stomach of insects. Could it similarly be damaging the integrity of our digestive tracts? The biotech companies insist that Bt-toxin doesn't bind or interact with the intestinal walls of mammals, and therefore humans. But here too they ignore peer-reviewed published evidence showing that Bt-toxin does bind with mouse small intestines and with intestinal tissue from rhesus monkeys. In the former study, they even found "changes in the electrophysiological properties" of the organ after the Bt-toxin came into contact.

If Bt-toxins were causing leaky gut syndrome in newborns, the passage of undigested foods and toxins into the blood from the intestines could be devastating. Scientists speculate that it may lead to autoimmune diseases and food allergies. Furthermore, since the blood-brain barrier is not developed in newborns, toxins may enter the brain causing serious cognitive problems. Some healthcare practitioners and scientists are convinced that this is the apparent mechanism for autism.

Thus, if Bt genes were colonizing the bacteria living in the digestive tract of North Americans, we might see an increase in gastrointestinal problems, autoimmune diseases, food allergies, and childhood learning disorders—since 1996 when Bt crops came on the market. Physicians have told me that they indeed are seeing such an increase." [xiii]

Bt-toxin is manufactured in every cell of a GM crop bred with it. There are entire blogs and websites dedicated to exposing the danger and harm caused by GMOs. Given the escalation in digestive problems, it's rather astounding that very few medical doctors will ever tell their patients to avoid GMOs and Roundup. Instead, the doctor will likely write a script for a pharmaceutical that won't fix anything and will likely cause side effects.

In another well-written article by Jeffrey Smith, titled "Are Genetically Modified Foods A Gut-Wrenching Combination?", he reported the following:

"The Bt-toxin produced by genetically modified corn kills insects by

punching holes in their digestive tracts, and a 2012 study confirmed that it punctures holes in human cells as well. Bt-toxin is present in every kernel of Bt corn, survives human digestion, and has been detected in the blood of 93% of pregnant women tested and 80% of their unborn fetuses. This "hole-punching toxin" may be a critical piece of the puzzle in understanding gluten-related disorders….

Bt-toxin may also activate the immune system. When mice were exposed to Bt-toxin, they not only mounted an immune response to it directly, but they subsequently reacted to foods that had not formerly triggered a response. There was something about the Bt-toxin that primed the immune system to become reactive to other, once benign, foods. If humans exposed to Bt-toxin react in a similar manner, eating GM corn could directly lead to the development of gluten or other food sensitivities.

Decreased digestive enzymes can create undigested food particles, contribute to the overgrowth of harmful bacteria, and promote symptoms of gluten-related disorders. Studies of mice eating Roundup Ready soy and fish exposed to glyphosate show that these compounds reduce digestive enzymes. All soybeans contain trypsin inhibitor, which blocks an important enzyme needed to digest protein, but Roundup Ready® soybeans contain as much as seven times more than non-GMO soy. The results of these studies suggest that genetically engineered foods may lead to serious digestive compromise." [xiii]

Chapter 6

INTESTINAL LANDMINE #4:

THE STANDARD AMERICAN DIET (SAD) &
BAD DIETARY HABITS

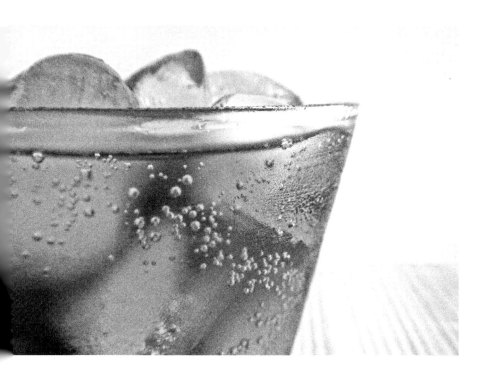

SODA, SPORTS DRINKS, AND BOTTLED BEVERAGES

Dehydration is a severe epidemic in the population. Your digestive system requires an adequate supply of water throughout the day to maintain proper intestinal homeostasis. Constipation plagues a significant percentage of people, and if there were a survey conducted on those with constipation and how much water they drink daily you would find that just about everyone afflicted isn't drinking enough. Soda doesn't hydrate the body, and neither do most bottled beverages. Dehydration freezes up the intestinal system.

When you add on all the chemical additives and artificial ingredients in these products, it makes the problem even worse. These ingredients alter your hydrochloric acid in unhealthy ways and damage intestinal flora. In 2014, a published study linked diet soda to damaged intestinal flora and increased diabetes risk.

"Now, a new study published in the journal Nature introduces a new idea: Diet sodas may alter our gut microbes in a way that increases the risk of metabolic diseases such as Type 2 diabetes — at least in some of us. In the paper, researchers at the Weizmann Institute of Science in Israel describe what happened when they fed zero-calorie sweeteners, including saccharin, aspartame, and sucralose, to mice. To our surprise,

[the mice] developed glucose intolerance,' Weizmann researcher Eran Elinav tells us…And how it's happening may be even more surprising. Their experiments showed that artificial sweeteners can alter the mix of bacteria in the guts of mice and people in a way that can lead some to become glucose intolerant." [xiv]

If you factor in the other artificial ingredients such as flavors, sweeteners, colors, emulsifiers, stabilizers, and preservatives, used in the bulk of these drinks they are causing widespread intestinal disorders.

JUNK FOOD

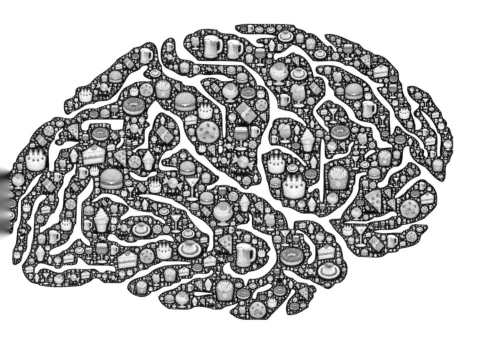

INVESTIGATOR'S REPORT

While few will admit it, the fact is our nation is hooked on junk food. These types of foods that make up most what people eat did not exist 100 years ago. Refined and processed foods consist of bread, pasta, breakfast cereals, refined flours, white rice, white sugar, chips, snacks, candy bars, packaged foods, and a slew of other food products that directly contribute this nation's diabetes, obesity and disease epidemic. Over time, eating enough of these will put you in a beautiful tomb with a shiny white headstone. Despite a century of evidence showing their ill effects on human health, studies indicate that they still make up roughly 30% of the average person's total carbohydrate intake each day. Approximately 90% of the average American's household food budget is spent on refined, processed foods; the majority of which are filled with additives and stripped of nutrients.

Most of these foods lack vital minerals and vitamins essential to good health while also lacking fiber and enzymes that are needed to break them down and process them through your digestive system. They have a two-fold damaging effect:

1.   They are causing severe nutrient deficiencies and pH imbalances.

2.   They are plugging up the intestinal system and turning your insides into concrete.

Fried foods can be added to the junk food category. Humanity was not designed to feast on three meals a day of meats and fried foods. Just about everything is being cooked in grease and oil, especially fast foods and restaurant meals. Fried foods are devoid of enzymes and full of toxins. This puts a severe strain on your digestive system because you are more than likely not obtaining these enzymes in sufficient quantity by consuming raw organic fruits and vegetables.

A typical day for someone starts like this: eggs and bacon for breakfast, burger or meat sandwich for lunch, afternoon snack, more meat for dinner. Everyone is born with a particular enzyme bank account when they are born. As we age, this account gets used up. When you factor in everything I have outlined in this report, it has a compounding effect that makes for a dangerous inflammatory situation.

MILK & DAIRY PRODUCTS

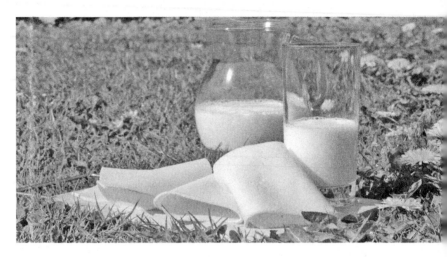

Linking dairy products to digestive problems is not difficult. For starters, a large percentage of the population lacks the necessary enzymes to digest milk and dairy products. Then you have to take into consideration that almost all dairy products have been pasteurized and homogenized. There's a big difference between a dairy cow raised to pasture on the grass in a fertile field that hasn't been treated with antibiotics versus a "factory farmed" dairy cow.

Factory farming typically confines the cows into crowded pens where they are treated with a genetically engineered hormone to produce more milk. The cows feast on a diet of genetically engineered grains, and the milk gets pasteurized after harvesting. However, pasteurization kills good and bad bacteria and enzymes needed by the body to process dairy. Pasteurization of dairy products began in the 1920's, and by 1950, it was commonplace. Organic sources of dairy products are pasteurized too. If you suffer from digestive distress, I will bet that you are a regular consumer of dairy products. If you want to correct your digestive condition, I would urge you to avoid all milk and dairy products for at least 30-days to see if you notice a difference.

Any imbalance, deficiency, or condition with your digestive/GI system triggers a breakdown in how your body metabolizes food and nutrients. Usually coupled with these problems are low enzymes, flora imbalance, the proliferation of harmful bacteria, low stomach acid, bloating, gas, chronic diarrhea, constipation, diverticulitis, acid reflux, celiac disease, gluten intolerance, etc. This then leads to the insufficient breakdown of proteins into its constituent parts – amino acids.

If your body cannot obtain all of the amino acids it needs from the diet, it will lead to a malfunction and breakdown in the production of hormones, chemicals, neurotransmitters, DNA, cell replication, and thousands of other bodily processes that all require amino acids and minerals to take place. The next domino that will fall is your immune system that requires the master anti-oxidant glutathione for regulation. The body builds glutathione.

However, it needs three amino acids to make that happen. Lack of amino acids will also cause problems with your liver because your body will not be able to detoxify efficiently enough. Your blood sugar can go haywire because insulin also requires amino acids for production.

Here's how critical this is. Did you know that even one deficient amino acid or mineral in the body can set up a cycle of disease? Any GI/Digestive disorder is a red flag that there is already an amino acid imbalance and mineral deficiency occurring. Lack of amino acids and minerals at the cell level are the two leading problems associated with virtually every disease known to man.

Chapter 7

HOW TO COUNTER IMPAIRED DIGESTIVE FUNCTION

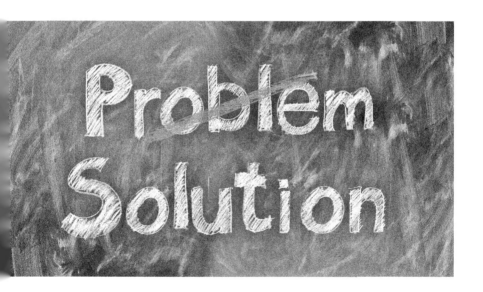

PROTOCOL #1 - USE SUPPLEMENTS THAT STIMULATE AND REPAIR THE DIGESTIVE SYSTEM

If you don't want to be counted in the digestive disorders statistics kept by the government, then it's time to take some proactive steps to turn things around. Using herbs and supplements to stimulate the colon and digestive system to remove toxins and unwanted fecal debris is imperative, especially if your diet consists mainly of refined carbohydrates, sugar, white flour, fried foods, milk and dairy products, processed meats, and restaurant foods.

It is essential that you monitor how often you go to the bathroom. For example, if you eat 2-3 meals per day and only go to the bathroom once a day, or worse, go days without at least one healthy bowel movement, that should be a clear indication that something must be done pronto. Time is of the essence before it cascades into a something far more severe.

Switching over to a healthier diet is a great place to start, although that is not always convenient or even practical for everyone. If you want to repair your digestive function, but you just don't think you can make a radical dietary change, at least follow my advice and start detoxing regularly and incorporating the other aspects I have outlined in this chapter. Our bodies were not designed to survive on the standard American diet (SAD) that passes off as food in Western society. It's time to get serious about digestive health before you end up with a severe disorder such as colon cancer that requires surgical removal of the cancerous part of the colon along with radiation and chemotherapy.

The body needs adequate fiber intake, water, fresh fruits and vegetables, nuts, grains and seeds, acid balancing minerals, probiotics, digestive enzymes, amino acids, chlorophyll, green foods, and fermented foods. The good news is supplement science can help you achieve all of this quickly and efficiently.

One of the most effective ways to begin the digestive restoration processes is to use a product called Temple Cleanse. This product has been on the market for over 15 years. Thousands of satisfied users have been able to restore digestive function by using this all-natural supplement. Unlike OTC stool softeners and herbal supplements that are not designed for long-term use, Temple Cleanse can be used daily for as long as you need it.

Temple Cleanse is one of the most gentle and effective constipation eliminators and digestive system restoration products being sold. The secret to its performance is a unique source of magnesium and oxygen. Oxygen is nature's most powerful cleansing agent, and in the digestive system, its ability to cleanse is second to none. Temple Cleanse contains a form of magnesium that holds stabilized oxygen molecules intact until it reaches your stomach acid. The acid releases the oxygen from the magnesium and disperses it throughout the entire digestive system for up to 12 hours or more.

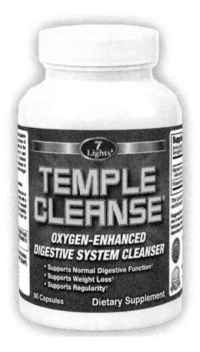

Available on Amazon

Glyphosate is a chemical pesticide, and Bt is a genetically engineered bacterial pesticide. If your digestive system is not working correctly and you are ingesting GMOs and glyphosate, you don't want these substances festering in your digestive system and wreaking havoc. You need to eliminate them. Temple Cleanse can help eradicate wastes and toxins that are stored in your digestive system and do wonders for gastrointestinal function.

Flora releases nascent oxygen in the digestive system which keeps aerobic bacteria thriving. With a malfunctioning gastrointestinal system, flora is crippled and cannot do its job correctly. This leads to the proliferation of anaerobic bacteria and other germs such as parasites that will put you on a fast track towards disease if not corrected. That is another reason why Temple Cleanse works so well. The dispersing of oxygen mimics healthy flora to help get your system functioning normally again.

If you suffer from constipation, bloating, gas, bowel irregularity, leaky gut, or just about any other digestive related issues, then you are a candidate for Temple Cleanse. Temple Cleanse helps to purge impacted wastes and cleanse the colon gently. Temple Cleanse causes no stomach cramps or discomfort either like some herbs and stool softeners. Temple Cleanse works by using oxygen and magnesium, which are very safe, gentle and effective.

Once Temple Cleanse your stomach the hydrochloric acid causes a natural chemical reaction to occur that separates the oxygen from the magnesium slowly and in a time-released manner.

This has a two-fold benefit. First, the form of magnesium used is designed explicitly to passes through the intestinal system and stimulate the bowels for the release of toxins and waste. Second, as the oxygen releases from the magnesium throughout this process, it loosens impacted waste and cleans up the stagnant debris.

The benefits of Temple Cleanse include:

- Eliminates Constipation in 24-Hours or Less
- Helps Alleviate Stomach Pain
- Helps Balance Stomach Acid and Stabilize pH
- Can Be Used Safely By Children and Adults
- Dramatically Improves Nutrient Absorption By Restoring Digestive Function
- Increases Intestinal Integrity and Flora
- Detoxifies Pesticides and Harmful Wastes Trapped In The Digestive System
- Helps Eliminate Gas, Bloating and Foul Odors
- Flattens The Stomach and Stimulates Weight Loss
- Supports the Entire Digestive System
- Improves Physical Wellbeing
- Reduces Tiredness and Relieves Insomnia Caused By Intes-

tinal Distress

- Non-toxic, Non-addictive, No Harmful Side Effects

PROTOCOL #2 - CORRECT NUTRITIONAL DEFICIENCIES CAUSED BY DIGESTIVE DISORDERS

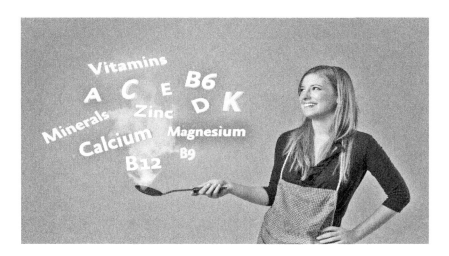

Any digestive related issue is a clear indication that your body is deficient in essential vitamins, minerals, amino acids, and phytonutrients. Your digestive system must be working optimally for nutrient transfer to take place, especially synthesizing amino acids from your protein intake. That's why in conjunction with Temple Cleanse, the next product I highly recommend is called Complete All-In-One by 7 Lights Nutrition. This cutting-edge nutraceutical is concentrated into an easy-mixing, excellent tasting berry flavored drink that is bursting with bioavailable nutrition that your cells crave.

Complete All-In-One delivers five blends of selected ingredients for healthy living, antioxidant protection, DNA support,
increased energy, immune support, digestive function, and much
more. Here is what you will find in this formula:

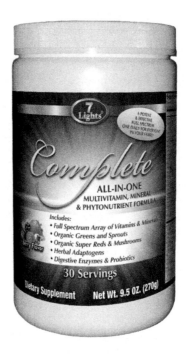

Available on Amazon

Blend #1: 35 Different Vitamins, Minerals & Amino Acids

Complete All-In-One goes above and beyond your basic one
daily. For starters, this product comes in a smooth mixing powder,
assuring rapid delivery of the nutrients. There is no need to break

down tablets or digest capsules which is not a smart way to go if you're trying to fix digestive related problems. Tablets are one of the worst delivery mechanisms for a multivitamin. It is a proven fact that absorption is hindered. Additionally, this product doesn't contain low-grade synthetic sources of vitamins and minerals that are poorly utilized. This product provides excellent bioavailability using the highest-grade natural vitamins and minerals that have scientific validation of their absorption potential in the body. It also combines amino acids which act as a protein source in the blood to help chaperone your nutrients into the cells.

Blend #2: Organic Super Greens & Sprouts

Wheatgrass, barley grass, chlorella, spirulina and many other dark green superfoods contain superior nutrients that can make a profound difference in your health. Not only are they chock full of plant-based vitamins and minerals, but they also provide the highest sources of chlorophyll you can find in foods. Greens assist in pH modulation, detoxification, digestion and nutrient assimilation. Complete All-In-One comes with a comprehensive blend of super greens that separates the formula from the rest of the competition.

Blend #3: Organic Super Reds & Mushrooms

Red foods are well known for their fantastic antioxidant protection that fight free radicals. Things such as beets, raspberries, and pomegranates, which you will find in this blend, have very high ORAC (Oxygen Radical Absorbance Capacity) scores that make them superior antioxidants.

Red foods are also great for:

- Boosting Energy Levels
- Supporting the Immune System
- Maintaining Health & Vitality
- Supporting Heart & Circulatory Health

Blend #4: Herbal Adaptogens

Adaptogens are natural substances that work with your body to help adapt to stress, fatigue, and low energy. Adaptogens work with regulating essential hormones and glands such as the adrenal. Our fast-paced lifestyles and poor dietary choices have caused widespread health challenges that often don't get addressed in your typical one daily. That's why we made it a point to include a comprehensive herbal adaptogen blend that combines clinically studied and proven herbs that can help the average person cope better given all of these challenges.

Adaptogens offer several other health benefits, including:

- Boosting the Immune System

- Supporting Healthy Weight

- Increased Physical Endurance and Mental Focus

- Reduction in Discomfort Caused by Poor Health

- Encouraging a Balanced Mood

Blend #5: Digestive Enzymes & Probiotics

Our digestive system works to digest food with digestive enzymes and other secretions, absorb nutrients and water and expel wastes and toxins. Most people are not getting enough live foods in their diet that provides adequate enzymes for digestion. Any multivitamin formula worth its price must include enzymes to aid in digestion and nutrient absorption. That's why this formula contains a digestive enzyme and a probiotic blend that you will not find in virtually any other one daily supplement.

Here are the supplement facts listing the ingredients:

Supplement Facts

Serving Size: 1 Scoop (9 g)
Servings Per Container 30

	Amount Per Serving	% DV
Calories	15	
Total Carbohydrate	3 g	1%*
Dietary Fiber	1 g	4%*
Vitamin A (as beta-carotene)	2,500 IU	50%
Vitamin C (as calcium ascorbate, acerola fruit extract & camu camu fruit extract)	300 mg	500%
Vitamin D (as cholecalciferol)	1,000 IU	250%
Vitamin E (as d-alpha-tocopheryl acetate & mixed tocopherols)	30 IU	100%
Vitamin K [as phytonadione (K1) & menaquinone (K2)]	100 mcg	125%
Thiamin (as thiamine HCl & benfotiamine)	15 mg	1,000%
Riboflavin (as riboflavin-5-phosphate)	11.9 mg	700%
Niacin (as inositol hexanicotinate)	20 mg	100%
Vitamin B6 (as pyridoxine HCl & pyridoxal-5-phosphate)	14.6 mg	730%
Folate [as (6S)-5-methyltetrahydrofolic acid, glucosamine salt]	400 mcg	100%
Vitamin B12 (as methylcobalamin)	150 mcg	2,500%
Biotin	300 mcg	100%
Pantothenic acid (as D-calcium pantothenate)	35 mg	350%
Calcium (as calcium citrate-malate)	220 mg	22%
Magnesium (as dimagnesium malate)	170 mg	43%
Zinc (as zinc bisglycinate chelate)	8 mg	53%
Selenium (as selenium amino acid chelate)	40 mcg	57%
Manganese (as manganese bisglycinate chelate)	1 mg	50%
Chromium (as chromium nicotinate glycinate chelate)	120 mcg	100%
Molybdenum (as molybdenum amino acid chelate)	42 mcg	56%
Sodium	45 mg	2%
MSM (methylsulfonylmethane)	250 mg	†
L-Glutamine	200 mg	†
N-Acetyl-L-cysteine	100 mg	†
Glycine	100 mg	†
Betaine HCl	100 mg	†
L-Lysine HCl	100 mg	†
N-Acetyl-L-tyrosine	75 mg	†
PABA	50 mg	†
Coenzyme Q10	50 mg	†
Alpha Lipoic acid	30 mg	†
Inositol	25 mg	†
Silica [from horsetail extract (aerial parts)]	20 mg	†
L-Alpha-Glycerylphosphorylcholine (GPC)	15 mg	†
Boron (as boron citrate)	1 mg	†

Organic Super Greens & Sprouts Blend: 1 g †

Wheat grass, green pea fiber, barley grass, blue green algae (spirulina), chlorella, green tea leaf, plum, orange peel, apple fiber, lemon peel, kale, broccoli, spinach, parsley, green cabbage, alfalfa grass, wheat grass, tomato, sweet potato, pumpkin, dandelion root, collard greens, dulse, adzuki sprout, amaranth sprout, buckwheat sprout, chia sprout, flax sprout, garbanzo bean sprout, lentil bean sprout, millet sprout, pumpkin sprout, quinoa sprout, sesame sprout, sunflower sprout

Organic Super Reds & Mushroom Blend: 1 g †

Beet, carrot, apple, blueberry, raspberry, strawberry, shitake mushroom, reishi mushroom, maitake mushroom, cherry, pomegranate, grape, peach, acai berry (Euterpe oleracea), banana, bilberry, goji berry (Lycium barbarum), black currant, elderberry, maqui berry, pineapple, papaya, blackberry, lemon, pear, cranberry, orange

Herbal Adaptogenic Blend: 500 mg †

Maca root, Panax ginseng root extract, Rhodiola rosea root extract, Gymnema sylvestre leaf, gynostemma leaf & stem extract, eleuthero root

Digestive Enzymes & Probiotic Blend (500 million CFU): 100 mg †

Fungal amylase, amyloglucosidase, cellulase, fungal protease, acid protease, lipase, Bacillus coagulans, Lactobacillus acidophilus, Lactobacillus casei, Bifidobacterium bifidum, Bifidobacterium longum, Lactobacillus rhamnosus, Streptococcus thermophilus

* Percent Daily Values (DV) are based on a 2,000 calorie diet.
† Daily value (DV) not established.

Other Ingredients: Guar Gum, Citric Acid, Natural Flavors, Organic Rebaudioside A, Organic Rice Hull Concentrate.

Keep out of reach of children.
Protect from heat, light and moisture.
Store at 15-30°C (59-86°F).
Do not purchase if seal is broken or missing.

Manufactured for:
7 Lights | Windermere, FL 34786
1.800.593.6273 | www.7Lights.net
© 2017 All Rights Reserved

TC# 3101690270

Protocol #3 - Take Amino Acid Supplements or Consume Foods That Supply Easily Digested Amino Acids To The Body

Any gastrointestinal disorder is a tell-tale sign of insufficient protein metabolism. If your body cannot break protein down effectively into amino acids, it is a guarantee that your health will suffer as a result. Every single biochemical, hormone, neurotransmitter, DNA, and cell process in your body requires a full spectrum blend of amino acids.

Glutathione is a tripeptide constructed from three amino acids – Glycine, Glutamic Acid, and Cysteine. Glutathione is considered the body's master antioxidant that disarms free radicals. Your body produces glutathione. If you suffer from digestive distress, it is a virtual guarantee that you are not efficiently breaking down your protein into all of the amino acids your body needs. This is why there is a direct correlation between immune system health and digestion. Poor diet and digestive problems along with pollution, heavy metals, toxins, viruses, bacteria, medications, stress, trauma, aging, infections, and even the normal aging process can all deplete your body's glutathione.

Proper amino acid supplementation may be an efficient way to restore healthy glutathione levels in the body. Proteins are large molecules that need to be broken down by the human body with enzymes before they can be absorbed and utilized within the cells.

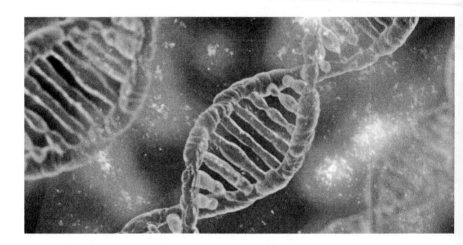

Leading practitioners are linking insufficient digestion and intestinal disorders to glutathione depletion. If your body is depleted of glutathione there is most likely a compromised immune system at play too. Any shortfall in just one essential amino acid can result in a degenerative medical condition. It's no wonder why immune system disorders are so prevalent today given the fact that the body's master antioxidant is not being produced sufficiently enough in the cells. An epidemic of gastro-intestinal disorders is depriving the body of essential amino acids it needs to build and repair.

Look for whole food derived sources of amino acids for best results. I recommend a product called Amazing Aminos which is derived from Norwegian salmon and is in a predigested state. Organically grown lean meats and fish in small quantities can help. Try avoiding lots of steaks, red meat, and conventional meats such as turkey, chicken and all pork, especially all fried meats and sausages, as these require lots of enzymes to process and are a proven strain on the body's digestive system.

Some better alternatives to a meat meal would be organic grass-fed whey protein, green food supplements (wheat grass, barley grass, spinach, spirulina, chlorella, etc.), Bragg's Liquid Aminos, hemp protein, plant-based proteins, sprouted beans and legumes, fermented tofu, and cultured organic yogurts.

Protocol #4 - Take A Full Spectrum Mineral Supplement Every Day

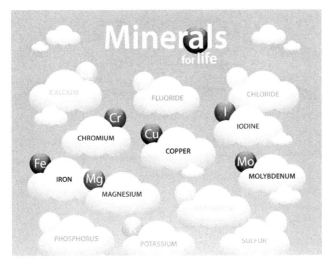

Minerals and amino acids are the two most important elements our bodies need every day along with water and oxygen. There are many ways to obtain the minerals your body needs. Unfortunately, most of what's sold on the market or contained in our foods don't cut it.

Minerals don't repair or fix digestive disorders; they provide your body with the raw materials it needs that it has become deficient in as a result. The overload of refined and processed foods and the intake of all the acid creating substances we are ingesting are causing massive mineral deficiencies. Glyphosate has been shown to disrupt the body's mineral balance. It is quite easy to make a connection to almost every disease known to man and a shortage of amino acids and minerals.

The most comprehensive and complete mineral supplement that I endorse is Living Stones. This is a foundational mineral formula explicitly designed to deliver all the critical minerals your cells need in a bio-available form that provides maximum cellular absorption. The primary minerals used are in amino acid chelated form produced by Albion Labs, which is the industry gold standard for mineral supplementation. This process allows the pure elemental mineral to make its way past the digestive system and into the blood. Since the amino acid, the mineral is bonded to is a food source, your cells allow it to enter unhindered, and they go to work almost instantly doing their job.

Living Stones is further enhanced with a copious amount of MSM (Organic Sulfur), a locomotive mineral that acts as a catalyst to pull minerals and nutrients into the cells. Most soils are deficient in sulfur and pesticides such as Roundup interfere with the sulfur cycle and kill off beneficial microbes needed to pull nutrients from the ground into the plants.

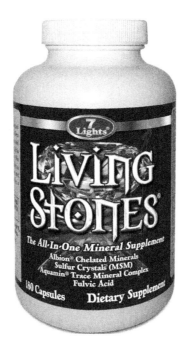

Available on Amazon

The blend is further enhanced with Aquamin, a unique ocean-based seaweed harvested off the coast of Ireland that provides a full spectrum array of over 74+ trace minerals. Seaweed extract is prized for its health benefits because these unique ocean plants contain a mineral profile in a matrix that almost mirrors the mineral profile of human blood plasma.

Last, but not least, Living Stones contains Shalijit. Shilajit has been reported to contain at least 85 minerals in ionic form, as well as triterpenes, humic acid and fulvic acid.

The primary active ingredients in Shilajit are fulvic acids, dibenzo alpha pyrones, humins, humic acids, trace minerals, vitamins A, B, C and P (citrines), phospholipids and polyphenol complexes, terpenoids. Also present are microelements (cobalt, nickel, copper, zinc, manganese, chrome, iron, magnesium and others. Shilajit comes from the Sanskrit compound word shilajatu meaning "rock-invincible", which is the regular Ayurveda term. [xv]

Protocol #5 - Use Other Supplements That Assist With Digestion

Many herbs assist with digestion that you can take in addition to some of the recommendations above. Ginger, cascara sagrada, dandelion, senna, curcumin, licorice, aloe, cayenne pepper, bitter herbs, activated charcoal, enzymes, probiotics, and essential oils (peppermint, orange, lemon, grapefruit) are just a few of the many well-known natural protocols that can help assist and repair digestive function.

Cycling probiotics several times throughout the year is not only a wise decision, but it is also necessary. If your symptoms have reached a chronic state, you will need to stay on a probiotic supplement every day. Look for supplements that have a wide range of strains in high quantity for best results.

Taking digestive enzymes with each meal is another wise investment given the fact that your digestion is already impaired. Drinking homemade fruit and vegetable juices and consuming more fermented foods such as sauerkraut, kombucha, pickles, miso, tempeh, and Natto, on a more frequent basis can all help provide enzymes to the body and cultivate a healthy digestive system. Green food supplements are tremendously beneficial for their cleansing and purifying abilities.

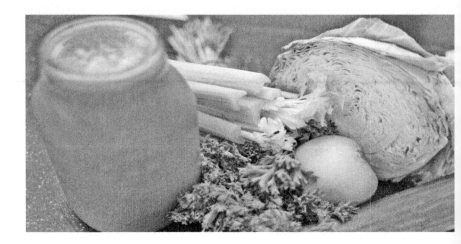

Essential oils are often never considered for digestion however, they can have a profound effect on digestive health. They can either be added to your water throughout the day or you can take empty capsules and fill them with essential oils and swallow them. There are many essential oils that can be ingested. The ones that have the best benefit on the digestive system are all derived from citrus fruit products.

Protocol #6 - Drink Organic Apple Cider Vinegar Every Day

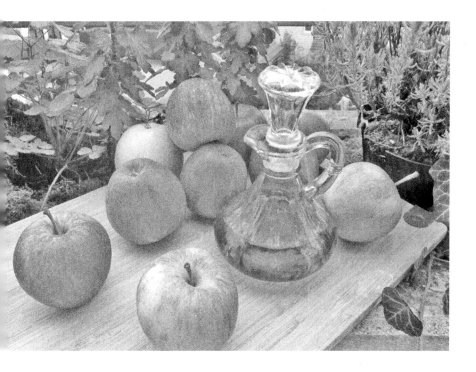

Mixing organic apple cider vinegar with 8-12 ounces of pure water and drinking it first thing in the morning and at least one more time later in the day may be one of the best decisions you ever made for your digestive system. Apple cider vinegar will do wonders for balancing stomach acidity, neutralizing acid reflux, eradicating heartburn, supporting enzyme function, and stimulating the bowels. I am shocked by the number of people I have consulted who tell me they never heard about drinking apple cider vinegar. Consider this a $5 elixir that will do more for your digestive related problems than any OTC antacid or prescription drug on the market. The best part of all is that you don't have to get ripped off on an expensive doctor visit only to get pushed into a costly prescription designed to supposedly "manage" your symptoms but will never fix and reverse your problems altogether. Spend the time researching on Google on the health benefits of apple cider vinegar. You will be astounded. There isn't a naturopathic doctor in the world that doesn't tout the benefits.

CONCLUSION

Thank you for taking the time to read this book. I hope the content has made you more aware of this topic. If you made it this far, I want to say congratulations. You are now more knowledgeable about the #1 medical problem facing our society than most people, including medical doctors. You have learned how prevalent digestive disorders have become, what some of the leading conditions are, what's causing the crisis, and what you can do to correct the problem.

Please support our work by sharing this book with others since you likely know family members, friends, and co-workers going through challenges with their digestion that just might be too embarrassed to seek answers.

[i] http://www.foxnews.com/health/2013/11/22/survey-shows-74-percent-americans-experience-gi-discomfort/

[ii] http://www.niddk.nih.gov/health-information/health-statistics/Pages/digestive-diseases-statistics-for-the-united-states.aspx

[iii] https://www.niddk.nih.gov/health-information/digestive-diseases/constipation/definition-facts

[iv] https://www.niddk.nih.gov/health-information/digestive-diseases/constipation/symptoms-causes

[v] https://www.niddk.nih.gov/health-information/digestive-diseases/acid-reflux-ger-gerd-adults

[vi] https://www.ncbi.nlm.nih.gov/pmc/articles/PMC5440529/

[vii] https://www.ncbi.nlm.nih.gov/pmc/articles/PMC4831151/

[viii] https://www.ncbi.nlm.nih.gov/pmc/articles/PMC4425030/

[ix] http://www.ncbi.nlm.nih.gov/pubmed/24678255

[x] https://www.naturalnews.com/2018-02-08-glyphosate-from-monsantos-roundup-decimates-microbes-in-soils-human-gut.html

[xi] https://www.ncbi.nlm.nih.gov/pmc/articles/PMC3945755/

[xii] http://www.responsibletechnology.org/posts/2011/05/

[xiii] http://responsibletechnology.org/glutenintroduction/

[xiv] http://www.npr.org/blogs/thesalt/2014/09/17/349270927/diet-soda-may-alter-our-gut-microbes-and-the-risk-of-diabetes

[xv] https://en.wikipedia.org/wiki/Shilajit

Printed in Great Britain
by Amazon